10 Day Water Fast to Reverse* Diabetes

by

Gianna Giavelli

Disclaimer: This book is for information only it should NOT be taken as medical advice. The author is not a physician. Consult your doctor before beginning any medical fasts or dietary changes.

Table of Contents

Preface

*By reverse I mean to put you on the road to reversing your illness, NOT that simply ten days will totally reverse diabetes. Thanks!

I am not a doctor. This is not medical advice. This is just my story and what I've learned. Please consult a physician before considering a fast or making any changes to your diet. I do know a little bit about water fasting. I've done it several times and this is the detailed journey I made in recovering from severe diabetes and the research behind why I believed it would be helpful for diabetes.

First off, a ten day water fast is NOT going to reverse your diabetes, but it's a great step to assist in reversing your diabetes. The reason why is because studies show that diabetes is a disease of eating too many carbohydrates without breaks over too long periods of time. It's a slow progression. The first step is your liver converts the extra fuel to fat (de-novo lipogenesis). It then pushes that fat out to the blood and says "here ya go". But when you have too much for your body to use, it begins stuffing it into the liver itself. Same with the pancreas. Too much fat from too many carbs? It stuffs into the pancreas. Now it can take ten, twenty, thirty years before that fat reaches a critical point and that's called non-alcoholic fatty liver disease, and eventually if it continues – cirrhosis of the liver. Eek! And the same thing happens to the pancreas – taken too long you get beta cell death and your ability to produce insulin goes down. You then become what is called a 1.5 diabetic.

So how do you reverse this? How do you get the fat out. I know I'll go on a low carb ketogenic diet. NOPE! Won't get the fat out!

What about just eating very few calories every day? NOPE! Won't get the fat out!

I'll excessive like a bunny like biggest loser TV show while eating next to nothing – NOPE! Won't get the fat out!

But there is good news, there IS a way to get the fat out. At least, a good amount of it. And that is water fasting. OMG just fast on water? If you're reading this book you probably already know a lot about water fasts and that many people do 30 day water fasts.   In this program, it's just 10 days. Because that makes it a bit less scary and a quicker goal to hit.

The critical research which underlies this was the finding that after 14 days of water fasting the liver had purged 80% of it's bound fat. That's tremendous. So should I do a 14 day water fast instead of ten. If you can go for it! But you'll still get a very positive effect from ten days.

But fasting is so hard, I'm just going to alternate day fast – that is to say fast every other day. NOPE! That wont drain your liver fat. And worse, my god you will be hungry. You see once the body switches to digesting itself hunger shuts off. Because it has food – YOU! This shutoff happens around day 4 of a fast. So when you fast for 4 days you are really torturing yourself. When you fast for ten days, days 5-10 are pretty easy.

Another thing you should know is, I'm not someone who hypes fasts or keto or sells products or anything like that. I'm someone who got terribly sick and the doctors weren't helping. So I do this to help others who are terribly sick. And stop the medical establishment idiocy from making them sicker.

So I'm going to tell you my story, why I think this approach is the best one for Diabetics to reverse their condition, and finally I'm going to lay out a whole bunch of things to make your fasting easier. I'll describe my fast day by day and what was happening so you can get a sense of it and not worry in your own fast. And by things I mean products that will help (regular stuff not my profit from it brands) and how to prepare everything for the fast. And most importantly **HOW TO END THE FAST.**

I should tell you I've spent probably more than five years reading hundreds of research articles, watching probably a thousand videos, really digging for answers. One thing that was clear was the American Diabetic Solution of adding MORE insulin was the exact opposite of what was needed.

My path to finding an answer wasn't so easy. I got sidetracked by the likes of veganism, Dr. McDougal Starch Solution, and Dr. Dean Ornish, And that creepy bald guy with no eyebrows. A lot of people are saying they have answers. I wasted another five years getting sicker and sicker trying out a lot of them.

My goal is only to help others not to make money. Jesus if I could have had this book two years ago it would have saved a lot of sick time and wasted life.

I want to thank Dr. Jason Fung for demonstrating that fasting reverses diabetes, Nina Teicholz for showing us the importance of meat and fat and unprocessed foods, and Dr. Benjamin Bikman for explaining the science of insulin and brown adipose tissue. These three people have changed the paradigm of diabetes treatment and lead me back to health. I highly recommend you watch every video they have on YouTube before you begin this fast.

I want to say again, beware the low fat-ists vegans: Dr. Barnard, Dr. McDougal, the bald guy. I can tell you personally I tried it and it failed horribly for me. I don't think they work with very sick diabetic patients and get recoveries they are more focused on average people.

Once again, this is a guide book, not health advice. You MUST consult with your doctor before beginning any fast. There are also centers where you can have a fully medically supervised fast.

- Gianna Giavelli, Austin TX, July 2019

Why did we GET SICK ?

Basically we got sick because of evolution. Our bodies just can't adapt as fast as we have changed what food we produce. We had this invention the plow. And it let us plant crops. And in Asia they learned how to harvest Rice. But remember Asians didn't go through the ice ages (only northern asians like those in Hokkaido and Harbin) so they didn't evolve the fasting or the put on fat during abundance as well as northern Europeans did.

Well anyways there was this new food – grain. Barley, wheat, so many grains. So that switched our hunter diet of meats and vegetables to more carbohydrate. And then in the modern world with sweets, muffins, and pastries and ice cream and pizza – to much more carbohydrate. Really it is slave food. Because it's cheap and in abundance. America produces tons and tons of grains because the government subsidizes it. And then it has to go somewhere so companies invent crackers, breakfast cereals, snacks and chips, etc.

Well all of that over time kills you. It leads to fatty liver, fatty pancreas, and eventually diabetes.

"Hepatic steatosis – the deposition of fat in the liver where it should not be, is consistently one of the most important markers of insulin resistance. The degree of insulin resistance is directly related to the amount of fat in the liver. Rising alanine transaminase levels, a blood marker of liver damage, in obese children are directly linked to insulin resistance and the development of type 2 diabetes. Even independent of obesity, severity of fatty liver correlates to pre-diabetes, insulin resistance and impairment of beta cell function. " – Dr. Jason Fung, https://idmprogram.com/fatty-liver-t2d-25/

So it's pretty simply why we get sick. And the solution is to do just the opposite – eat none of that stuff anymore. Ever. Well I do a cheat day on the first of the month. But other than that, it's really a never again.

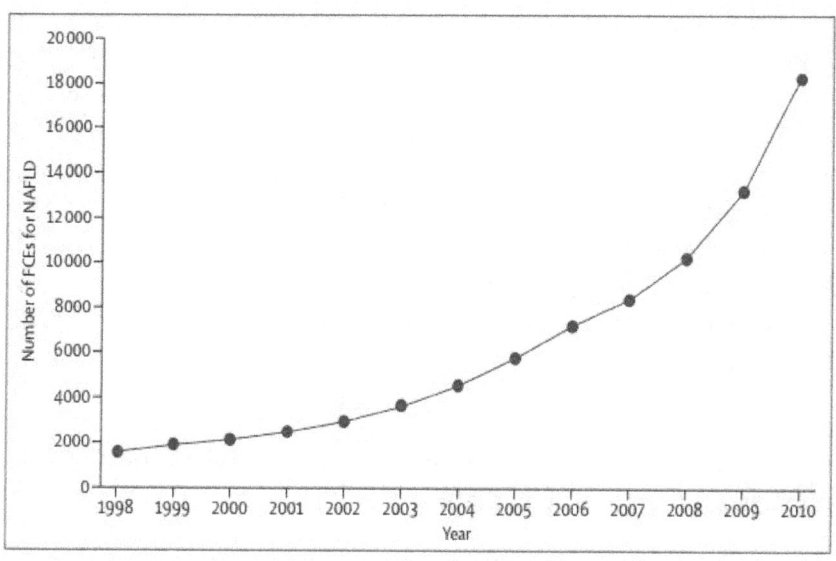

Figure 8: Number of hospital admissions for non-alcoholic fatty liver disease, 1998–2010
Admissions to hospital defined as first finished consultant episodes. Data are from Hospital Episode Statistics.[64] FCE=finished consultant episodes. NAFLD=non-alcoholic fatty liver disease.

You see diabetes is really (at least a large part of it) a disease of NAFLD (non alcoholic fatty liver) combined with fatty pancreas. And it's an epidemic.

Right now, you will look at that delicious frosted cupcake and go yum. But I swear, after the fast, your taste will totally change. And if you put your body on that meats and veggies and good fats (butter, tallow, bacon fat, suet, and maybe a tiny bit of coconut oil and a tiny bit of olive oil only on salads), the next time you look at that frosted muffin you won't crave it. You might even feel a bit ill about the though of eating it.

Grains were never our diet. Its the slave diet. The upper class would stay on their high meat diets, and the poor couldn't afford it. Italians, who were mostly quite poor, came up with so many foods based on grains – all kinds of pastas made of wheat, all kinds of cakes, and of course Pizza. As an Italian, trust me it sucks. My entire ethnic cuisine has been taken.

"Fatty liver precedes the diabetes diagnosis often by ten years or more. The emergence of the metabolic syndrome follows a consistent sequence. Weight gain, even as little as 2 kilograms (4.4 pounds) is the first detectable abnormality, followed by low HDL cholesterol levels. High blood pressure, fatty liver, and high triglycerides emerge next, at roughly the same time. The very last symptom to appear was the high blood sugars. This is a late finding in metabolic syndrome.

The West of Scotland study confirmed that fatty liver and elevated triglycerides precedes the diagnosis of type 2 diabetes by at least 18 months. The triglyceride level increased more than 6 months before the diagnosis. This is strong evidence that accumulation of liver fat is crucial to the development of insulin resistance, but also may act as a trigger for the development of

type 2 diabetes." -Dr. Jason Fung,
https://idmprogram.com/fatty-liver-t2d-25/

There are also studies where people had massive liposuction, but there was change in their high glucose levels. It's not Bag4 fat, it's organ fat. And that only comes out during a multi-day fast.

Living without carbs is hard to sustain long term, but there have been a few substitutes that have gotten better over the years. Wish special mixes you'll be able to get a decent pancake or waffle with sugar free syrup. The first stuff was crap. But competition to make good versions has finally paid off and now you can get OK replacements. Will it ever be as good as the original. No, but it will be good enough to add some diversity to your new diet.

I should mention that the diet to be on is called the KETO DIET. And unlike when I did Atkins and ate special bars, tons of cheese and shrimp, and lots of steaks, this is different. This diet is 5% of your calories from carbs, 30% from protein, and 65% from fat. Fat fat fat. Why? Its the energy source which does not spike your diabetics and blood sugar. So you become a fat eater.

But there is another advantage with the KETO diet – you naturally exclude grains especially WHEAT which, if you've developed NAFLD and diabetes you probably are one of the 1 in 3 americans who have issues with grains and didn't know it. So KETO eating, while we think the advantage of it is simply low carb to burn off our fat and lose weight, actually another quite beneficial aspect of it is that you've STOPPED POISONING

YOURSELF WITH GRAINS. Strong words? Diabetes leads to blindless, kidney failure, amputation and death. Not strong enough words I think.

With just enough low carb vegetables – spinach, mushroom, pepper, cauliflower – to keep you sane. For example, my breakfast might be 2 free range eggs with 1/3 cup of heavy cream cooked In bacon fat with some fresh cooked baby spinach leaves on the side. Tastes great. Or a chili with ground beef (grass fed free range) and with Anaheim peppers and a few Goya black beans and fire roasted tomatoes. Sure, I'd love to add corn to the chili but that's a starchy veg so it gets kicked. Instead I eat it with a good organic expensive sour cream. Yum. Can't complain about that and the spices give it a good kick to make you feel like its real food. I use a InstantPot type thing, and just sear the beef first then set it to 30 minutes of pressure cooking with all the ingredients and spices in. It's real easy to make. And fish you can eat fish. I like raw fishes like oysters, or oysters Rockefeller, and shrimp cocktails, or go to a sushi place and get sashimi (ugh what a waste of money, just by the fish and do a at home sashimi!). The point is, KETO eating is tough but not impossible. And when you get that choice high grade grass fed T-Bone or porterhouse steak on the grill with a side of grilled asparagus its tough to feel like you are being slighted.

So to recap – grains are poison to you as a diabetic. You have to cut them cold turkey. FINITO! NO MORE! (except when you are a lot further down the path to health you might add the one day a month cheat. I use it to get a croissant in.).

Also off the list of eating are starchy veggies – corn, potatoes, squashes. Yes even sweet potatoes. Beets. All starchy veggies are FINITO. NO MORE.

Avoid nuts, but you can have a few walnuts or macadamia nuts once a day.

So once you finish the fast, you go on by eating KETO foods. There's ton of information on what is a good KETO food and what is banned on the web.

Now just eating KETO might NOT lead to weight loss like it does in healthy people. So then you have to introduce a number of fasting days. Maybe just one a week, maybe two. Until you see the scale moving down every week. Once you are in the right direction stick with it, and when you get closer to your goal weight, you've probably regained enough insulin production to run your body just fine, but keep the poison carbs away. Use your renewed health for a few cheats of the old tastes or you'll end up right back where you started.

Insulin was NEVER the answer

Doctors are obsessed with the blood glucose level, but never the insulin level. But diabetes is a disease of HIGH insulin and insulin resistance. Dr. Fung tells us why Insulin isn't the answer.

"Your doctor may prescribe a medication such as insulin injections, or perhaps a drug called Metformin, to lower blood glucose, but *these drugs do not rid the body of excess glucose.* Instead, they simply continue to take the glucose out of the blood and ram it back into the body. It then gets shipped out to other organs, such as the kidneys, the nerves, the eyes, and the heart, where it can eventually create other problems. The underlying problem, of course, is unchanged." Dr. Jason Fung, The Diabetes Code.

In fact, I like to think of insulin like a bicycle pump for glucose. The cell is saying "I'm bloated I can't take anymore!" so you push the pump and increase the pressure and go "TAKE MORE TAKE MORE" if the cell doesn't, a few more pumps and the pressure goes even higher. This eventually results in kidney failure, vision problems, liver failure, and eventually loss of mortality (aka death). Fung calls it the overstuffed suitcase, but I like the bicycle pump. We've all pumped up a bicycle tire too high and heard it burst (well if you were a racing cyclist like I used to be in college you have!). That's really what's happening when you take Insulin. Metformin is just a proxy to stimulate the liver to signal to produce more insulin. So they are about the same.

The problem is your body is literally packed with glucose after years of insulin resistance – worse if you actually take supplemental insulin. Taking supplemental insulin IS REQUIRED for people who refuse to fast or change their diets. But it's not a cure. It just speeds up death and dysfunction while giving doctors their perfect blood glucose results.

Fung likes to say "the BLOOD GLUCOSE got better with insulin, but the diabetes got worse" that's a very telling statement. It's as if doctors are looking at the wrong thing altogether. Why would they continue to make that mistake?

Well insulin is very expensive. And all the testing and monitoring equipment and blood tests from labs all cost billions. They don't want things to change. It's big money.

Worse, multiple studies show that insulin and Metformin treatment for diabetics do no slow or reduce the incidence of heart disease and cardiac death in diabetic patients. Stew on that for a minute. The glucose remains, so your body rots, your organs rot and you die.

So HOW do you get the glucose OUT without medications which did nothing to get the glucose out?

First answer is don't put it in. That's where very low carbohydrate dieting and KETO eating comes into play. BUT if you are in sick mode, that isn't going to get you there, not fast enough to recover. You need to do something a bit more .. which is to reduce carbohydrates AND protein which causes insulin load to ZERO. You see even fat and protein cause SOME insulin secretion and if you are in a hyper insulin resistant state, well any eating at all is still going to produce insulin which is going to BLOCK glucose release and the insulin then BLOCKS your brown adipose tissue from burning off excess glucose (by generating heat).

So how do you get these numbers to zero so your insulin levels go down and your BODY GLUCOSE starts to filter OUT of all the nooks and crannies where it's been packed in over 20 years?

Answer: YOU FAST

And it's the only answer really. Yes low carb eating and hyper exercising can eventually clear out BODY GLUCOSE but you'd feel so terrible it's doubtful you could do it. And most diabetic patients are older as it's a progressive disease (although this is now horrifically changing as now even Teens who gorge on sugar and carbs all day long are developing type 2 diabetes before the age of 18. That used to be considered impossible but its a sad statement on how sick our societies diet has become) – so these older patients who are weak from high glucose really aren't going to go out and run five miles a day. So the answer is ... YOU FAST. How do I do that? Won't it be horrible? That's exactly where this book comes in. Read on my padawan, I will take you through EVERYTHING you need to know about fasting and how to make it as painless and easy as possible, what to do, how to prepare, and most importantly what NOT TO DO. Both what not to do during a fast, but also what not to do when breaking the fast and after the fast.

Fasting has been a traditional remedy for centuries. One reason why fasting is so powerful is because Humans have the fasting ability built in. Our growing up and evolving in cold climates made us REQUIRE a fasting mechanism, to go into a ketogenic mode with higher adrenalin to get us through those lean times, and then recognize when food returns. Oddly enough, Chimps who evolved in equatorial Africa where there is no winter, lack the ability to fast.

When you fast your body goes into an amazing mode. It scavenges for faulty cells and consumes them (autophagy) and this can even help with cancer, but really its a whole body fix up. And one of the most important things it can do is to get the hard to remove ORGAN FAT OUT. Principally the liver, but also the pancreas. You'll hear me harp on that theme over and over. Because really that's one of the most important things to understand. If you used conventional dieting, you'd have to clear all your external body fat first, then your muscle fats, then your interstitial fats, before you'd get rid of a drop of organ fat. "Look I've lost 40 pounds!" but your organs are still sick with fat.

Fasting is different. It does get the organs to flush fat. The liver senses the low glucose levels and that triggers it to start breaking down the fat stores which have become damaging to the liver. If you haven't reached the stage called cirhosis then you have a good chance of recovery.

A lot of people especially Americans are TERRIFIED of not eating. YOU MUST EAT they exclaim over and over. But you don't. Your body is designed NOT to eat. In fact, a nice woman at work was so freaked out that I wasn't eating that I broke my fast early. OK I was also starting to get 2 signs that I should break my fast soon (I'll tell you what to look for) so it wasn't like I should just listen to her, but the HYSTERIA in her voice, a mom trying to save a dying child, well it was shocking to me. But that's the attitude.

So we eat, and worse, we snack late into the night, then eat first thing in the morning, then snack then eat more. All of this causes NO PERIOD OF REST FOR THE PANCREAS. This lack of a rest period is one reason why we get built up organ fats. Your body was designed for downtime when that fat could release, when your insulin would go low.

So you can see that injecting insulin is exactly the wrong thing you should be doing. Shocking, the American Diabetes Association strongly promotes taking insulin in REFUTATION OF THE RESEARCH and ALSO strongly advises AGAinST FASTING!

Yehp. Do they have any proof or research on their side showing reversal of diabetes with THEIR method? Nope. Nada.

During the 1950s there was this almost scientific mania that with the new chemistry and pills we could cure any disease. And sadly American medicine is stuck solidly in this paradigm. Pills and surgery. Cut out things if they arn't working great. Too fat? Take the stomach out. What if they took our hearts out at the first sign of heart disease? Thats nuts of course, but thats the American medical establishment's mindset.

Has their treatments worked? No if you look at the numbers. Diabetes is on the rise and once in the medical systems clutches patients go in, and don't come out.

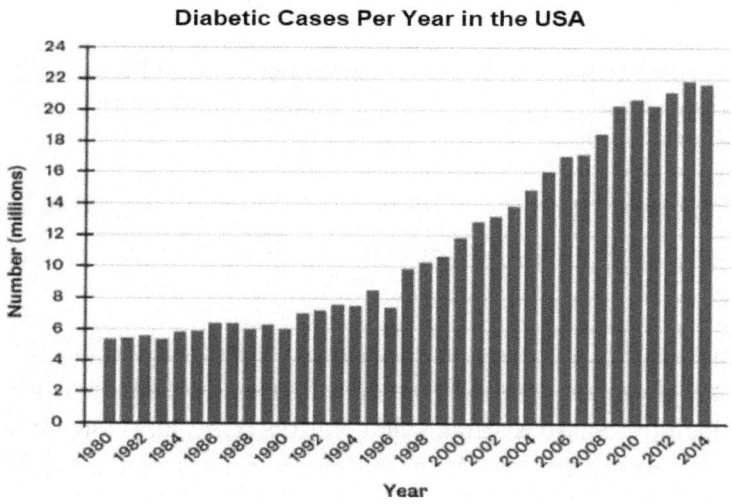

Diabetic Cases Per Year in the USA

That's exactly why I wrote this book. There was a lot of information on the new research and the new goal of fasting and keto to treat diabetes, but precious little information on how to fast and how to succeed on a fast targeted to diabetic patients. Read on I'm here to help!

An Epidemic of Wheat Intolerance and the Gliadin – Thyroid Disease Connection

One reason why I probably developed Grave's Disease (where your thyroid goes nuts and overproduces Thyroxine) is because I ate wheat and other gluten containing grains for years. It was the staple of the new American Diet thanks to the nutters who forged their research in the 60s and 70s. Liars like Ancel Keyes. Remember that food pyramid with 20 servings of grains and breads on the bottom? That was a death sentence for millions of Americans. And they STILL refuse to change the guidelines even though it's proven it's based on false research.

Well it seems that Gluten, if it can get through your intestines and into your bloodstream, which almost always happens on the intestine damaging grain diet, the gliadin molecule gets recognized by our body and attacked with antibodies as an invader. That's great, exactly what it should do. (sheez what a awkward run on sentence. Forgive me!)

Unfortunately our antibodies aren't soo exact as you might expect and they also recognize the Thyroid as an invader. So they begin to attack that as well. The antibody reaction is so strong that if you eat ONE PIECE OF BREAD your thyroid would get attacked non-stop for SIX months. Well that's what happened to me. So going keto and grain free is a good idea for the thyroid connection as much as it is for general health or weight loss or diabetic treatment.

Dr. Ken Fine's discovered that **1 in 3 Americans** are gluten intolerant, and that **8 in 10** are genetically predisposed to gluten intolerance.

"We have **altered the wheat so much**, through hybridization and seed selection, to have more gluten and to be more favorable for farming practices, that we have to look at what gluten is ...... a highly antigenic food. It always has been. The coeliac affection was first described in 100 AD. So if we've been eating wheat, or grains, for 10, 000 years, then 8,000 years into this, gluten induced disease was written about, it was probably present long before that. The bottom line is that this is a 10,000 year old food with a 2000 year old description, so this is not a new syndrome.

What could be new is that because we have hospitals and tests the resulting diseases can now be identified earlier. Before you had to be near death before anyone knew there was anything wrong with you. But we are certainly able to identify celiac disease before you are dying from it.

I really think we are seeing more of an epidemic of non-celiac GS because, I believe, our immune systems are much more reactive than ever before. All autoimmune and immune diseases are on the rise. That's a fact from the NIH. The NIH has even acknowledged that there is probably an environmental component to that increase, and I agree with them. The wheat we grow now is more immune stimulating. The way I see wheat today is that it has become the poison ivy of the western diet."

There is one other food sensitivity diabetic connection which is that recent studies suggest that COWS MILK (non human milk) may be the cause of the immune reaction that leads to Type 1 Diabetes (total destruction of pancreatic beta cells). Ouch! So you may want to avoid cows milk (which is full of sugar anyways) and stick to no milk or almond milk especially for children.

So wheat and grains can lead to thyroid destruction which then leads to diabetes. Yehp. The non-thyroid path to diabetes seems to be mostly based on high carb and high sugar diets, and the longer hours of eating with lesser hours of downtime between meals. We are a nation of snack-ers and you can see the diabetic horror brewing in every big belly you see at Walmart.
Remember the liver gets fat FIRST so they certainly are on the path to doom.

The Double Whammy – Insulin and Brown Adipose Tissue

One reason I got fat was the double whammy. To understand the double whammy you have to first look at what happens with healthy thin people who have low insulin and functioning thyroid. Step one is simple, they eat a too big meal with way too many carbohydrates. Now calories in calories out says... oh they will put on fat. But not so fast. You see they have two secret mechanisms to fight back. The first mechanism is their brown adipose tissue which is in that interstitial abdominal fat. When it senses high levels of glucose in the blood, it literal switches on the HEAT. It literally burns it off and generates heat. Which is why sometimes people feel warm and sweaty after eating a gigantic meal and others overeat a ton of food and are skinny.

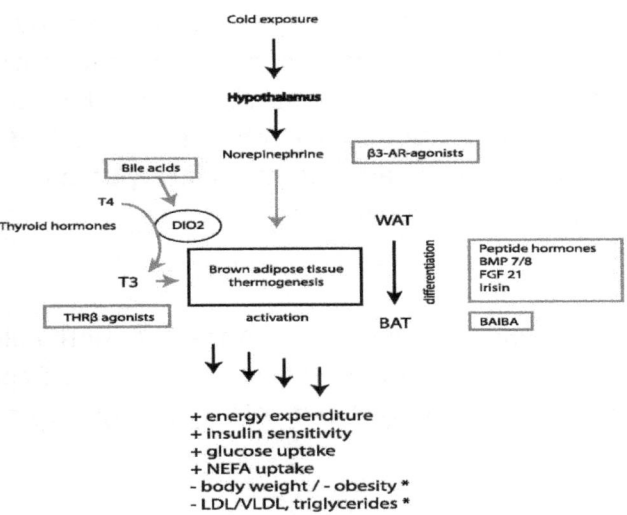

The sorry side of this for people like me is that high insulin SHUTS THIS DOWN (see Dr. Bikman's lectures on insulin) so the brown adipose cannot shift into generate heat and waste glucose calories to prevent the need to store it after a too big meal. So that with insulin we don't have this glucose to heat pathway. But that's ok because the healthy person has one other solution, which is to secrete MORE thyroid in response to a large meal. Again it revs metabolism across the body and the whole body burns off excessive glucose.

Back to my sorry state, my thyroid was killed by western doctors. I take pills in a set amount to generate my thyroid so it never responds to glucose big meals or too much carbohydrate intake. This is why thyroid patients who have had surgical removal or radiation treatment really are put on a path to diabetes without them knowing it.

Year after year the fat will increase in the liver until failure. The treatment is to add fasting to your diet, so you can correct on some days the fat that was put into your organs on normal eating days.

What is the protocol I'm using to get back to health?

One of the annoying things is a lot of the doctors who build a practice treating diabetics with fasting stay very tight lipped on what exactly their protocol is. So you have to go in and spend a lot of money. I'm not saying thatch a bad thing, and as I had NO associated good docs in my city (thatch pretty common all you have is the jab em full of insulin docs) I had to research it out.

So I read a lot of articles. I really dug in. And this is what seems to be the best. If you are healthy enough to do it. If you are frail or have heart conditions or other issues (check with your doctor I am not giving health advice!) then you may need to do a less aggressive approach.

So right away here it is:

Step 1: 10 Day Water Fast

During this stage your liver and pancreas fat flushes out and you begin to regenerate. Shorter fasts don't do that. Added In bone broth towards the end of the fast so its not just water. Please do not stop here and start a water fast - you must continue to read the rest of this book or you might get horribly sick. The 10 (or 14) day water fast is simply a good technique with lower risk than the 30 day fast. And it can be repeated as needed. I find I don't really lose weight at all even in a ketogenic state, so for me, it's a series of 10 day water fasts to get the weight down, losing about 8 to 10 pounds each time after re-feeding.

Step 2: Post Fast

Post fast is a low carb healthy fat diet (LCHF). The trick is not to gobble meat and get in good natural fats as well as great veggies like broccoli, spinach, cauliflower every day. Now if this doesn't continue to produce weight loss then you have to add in fast days. Up to three days a week of no eating. For example, Mon Fast, suet eat. Weds fast, Thurs eat Friday eat , sat fast and Sunday eat. Continue to weight goal. Personally I find these no eat days quite difficult and really I prefer the longer fasts. But it varies from person to person what works best for you.

That's it. And there's nothing stopping you from doing another 10 day fast or as you get more experienced fasting a 15 day fast. It might take a few times to get all that fat out of the liver. Cost to do it? Maybe 40 bucks in supplies and the price of good water. Well of course doctors can't make a living on that. But they'll still get you for office visits and blood work. God bless them.

One thing that makes this book different is I lay out exactly how to get ready for the fast, what to buy, all the things that will help you get through it as painlessly as possible. And it comes from being there doing it. I hope it helps people. So now that we've done the prelims, onward to my tragic story....

Getting Sick

The first big event happened in my twenties. Current research suggests it happened because I ate bread. Yep bread.
Apparently some of the gliadin molecule from bread slipped into my bloodstream and my body had a immune response to it. Unfortunately, the thyroid molecules are almost exactly the same. So my body started attacking my Thyroid gland. The result was it began to overproduce like crazy. My resting heart beat went to 180, I would get weak, and I became a skeleton.

I tried the two anti thyroid mess but I was allergic to one. Made me ferociously itch. So after three or so years on medical therapies, I caved and went for radiation treatment to kill the thyroid. That's a very western concept... if it's broken KILL IT or YANK IT OUT. Now why they couldn't calculate a series of smaller doses and just hit my thyroid several times until it's output went to normal. The answer is in our hurried western system they don't want to deal with it. Had I known what I did at the time I could have cut all grains from my diet and I might have gotten better. Not sure but ... maybe. So well they hamfisted killed my thyroid with six curies of fun in a little pill. My pee was radioactive for 24 hours which was kinda cool.

After that, they put me on synthroid which I got horribly sick on, then levoxyl which I got horribly sick on. You see to patent their drug, they ALTER the thyroid molecule from its natural form and usually stick on a carboxyl group somewhere. The other problem is their drug only has a form of T4. Not T3, T2, T1, or thyroid binding globulin molecule. I think that's what it's called. So I got really sick until I started digging on this new thing called the internet and found out about natural thyroid from pigs and cows. It had all the molecules and it wasn't altered. So I took that and I got better, but I noticed I was still quite weak in the morning. So we added T3 which is like crack cocaine basically, just a speck in the morning and again in the afternoon. It hits in about half an hour and the first thing is your heart races because it has a direct effect on coronary tissue. Well I had about figured it out, but I couldn't ever take enough medicine to get into the upper ranges. My legs would shake vigorously from the meds and keep me from sleeping. So I was stuck at the low end of normal. Which of course meant I got fat.

I worked in tech which meant long hours. Long intensive brain use. That led to being hungry well into the night and needing to snack. And mostly on carbs. I had tried low carb high fat dieting but never could stay on it more than three months. Takes a lot of will power to be carbless. I think a lot of people find that.

So the long and short of it was I put on about ten pounds a year, not much. But go forward 25 years and I was fat. Belly had bulged out past my boobs. My thighs rubbed together. Somehow the brain is good at MASKING this and hiding it from you. You really can't see you are fat. Don't ask me why but it's quite the same as the syndrome where men suck in their massive beer bellies and think they are charles atlas. There's just something programmed in our brains that make it hard for us to see our bodies falling apart with fat. And good ol Mr. Diabetes was waiting for me. My first symptoms were just weakness. We detected the high glucose at the docs and tried metformin. But the metformin knocked me way out. I tried to keep taking some but eventually gave up. My fasting glucose was in the 180s. A few years later it would skyrocket. I had a hard time using the glucose meter. I couldn't stick myself. So I didn't monitor things so carefully.

I had been working on my own company and research and working hard. I wasn't taking any thyroid meds because I didn't have health insurance so the cost to see the doc was high. Then I got a job and worked insanely hard for six months. I did eat well and healthy. Whole foods, grass fed beef, organic milk and butter. Vegetables. And few junk items. No sugar. I thought I was doing good. But it wasn't enough. After a while I had my first big sick. I had dropped my weight 20 pounds and I thought I was making good progress. But I wasn't. I didn't understand anything at all how this disease works and traps you.

When the first big sick happened I thought it was the flu because I was coughing horrible. It might have been the flu, but with a diabetic high glucose kick on top. I was in a state of extreme thirst and extreme peeing just a few drops every five minutes. But the urge to pee was overwhelming. So I couldn't sleep. And the craziest symptom, I couldn't eat. I finally found I could eat a cold crisp apple. It was the only thing I could have an appetite for. So there I was on one apple a day for two weeks. Finally I pulled out of it. I was still weak, tired. I couldn't clean the house.

I just wanted to mention that I was getting one diabetic symptom that scared me a lot. My feet were going numb. It was getting hard to walk. One foot was in trouble and then the other foot started to get bad. If both got bad, I would be reduced to stumbling. (PQQ can help with this, see the chapter – Pills I take every day)

Once I was back up and at it a little bit I tried to get my thyroid meds refilled. There was a walk in clinic by the grocery store where I got my waters. I had to drink very special water. American water seemed to have bleach in it and my body couldn't process it. I would drink gallons of the stuff and be in deep thirst. In the end it was two waters that sustained me. One the higher mineralized Topo Chico. And the other a less minerally Mineraga. Both Mexican products. Perrier was too bitter. Anyhew I went to the clinic and my good luck was able to see the I think it was a doctor the same day. Now normally before giving out thyroid meds, they run a thyroid panel and make sure you are deficient. But they wanted to run 300 dollars of extra blood tests. I tried to explain that they would be meaningless because my thyroid was out. But like a sucker I paid over $300 hoping to get a real 3 month script for meds. I even took in the old script, printed out by the pharmacy, so they could see it was what I had been on for years. They gave me a script for seven days and had a follow up doctors appt in fourteen days. What the hell? I went back in and told them they had gotten the script wrong and to please refill it. Nope, they never did. Then the phone calls started. Frantic phone calls. My labs had come in terrible. Sure my thyroid was was too low, but I had pissed out tons of things and a lot of metabolites were too low. And then came the reason they were freaking out. I had had a tiny cup of tomato soup that day. It probably had sugar in it. Bastards. I should have known I can't ever eat out. But that little tiny few spoon fulls of soup had pushed my glucose way up. Not quite a fasting measure. But in the super scary range. So they never gave me my script for thyroid even after all the money I paid and Immediately tried to send me to the vultures – the American Diabetic Association. They lined up a doctor for me and they started calling and they walk in place started calling. I posted a message that with my thyroid meds everything was getting better and p.s. Thanks for nearly killing me by not giving me my thyroid meds. I called my old place and set up to see the doc and they gave me a one month script. Ok that's covered and it would def help. But the high glucose. Holy jimminy I was sick! It was the day that came that I just didn't expect and wasn't quite ready for. It was the day I had to take radical intervention into my life. No more focus on work. This was serious and I was going to do something.

Luckily I knew what to do. I had done tons of research. I had seen Dr. Jason Fung reverse diabetes through fasting even in older more fail patients. If they can do it so can I I thought! I read the science behind it (which I'll get into shortly). And to be honest, he was one of the only ones reversing diabetes in really sick patients. Unfortunately, before I got to dr. Fung, I got side tracked by Dr. John "just eat lots of starch" McDougal and also by the creepy hairless guy – just eat fruit. He and his partner were Type I diabetics so they were in a somewhat different world. But it was easy to fall into their traps. I'm sure it does work for some people, but I was sick and when I tried their approaches, I got SICKER.

So I was stuck with a doctor's appointment coming up and in a terrible state. It was time to unleash the plan and start immediately. I began a 10 day water only fast. If I felt fine I would continue it out to 14 days.

Why 10 day fast and not alternate day fasting?

The first thing I want to say is when you do the 10 day fast you ONLY HAVE TO DO IT ONCE. Ok, you may CHOOSE to do another 10 day fast later if you really have a lot of weight to loose – like over 80 pounds. But after the fast you can switch to a slower gradual technique.

The first reason for 10 days and not 30 days is that it has been shown to be a pretty safe period of time to fast. People have fasted for 380 days. But many many people do 30 day fasts with no issues whatsoever. So it's a well established protocol. Of course if you are frail and have other medical conditions it might not be for you. But basically if your just fighting diabetes its just about perfect.

Just keep telling yourself – I ONLY HAVE TO DO THIS ONCE. Doesn't that make it seem a lot more achievable?

The American diabetes association thinks you can't do it. Officially "we don't recommend fasting" yah, they recommend drugs to make you sicker and fatter and eventually kill you.

Let me tell you my grandmothers story. They had her pumped full of insulin until she became a beach ball shape. Then she had a heart attack. Then they cut her leg off. Then she died. Take insulin? Not on your life. The PROBLEM is too high insulin.

Why not longer water fasts?

You will hear of 30 day water fasts. There have been deaths at several of the clinics that offer this service. People mostly who did too much activity during or after, or didn't refeed correctly, or didn't use bone broth and had the phosphorous issue (see below). From a safety standpoint 10 days is just a lot safer, your aren't going so deep into your reserves, and metabolic rate does not drop so much. Your base metabolic rate recovery after a fast can take some time. On a 10 day fast it has only dropped to around 90% so you won't run into the Biggest Loser syndrome (a TV show competition for weight loss) where the BMRs were so destroyed they went right back to fat after loosing a hundred pounds.

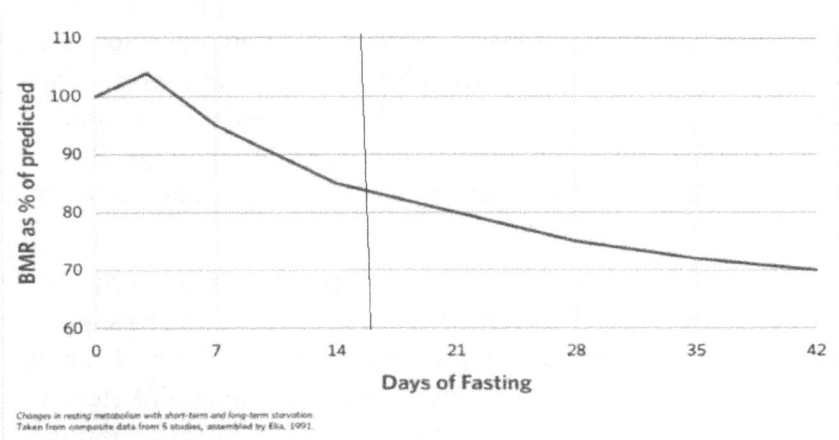

Changes in resting metabolism with short-term and long-term starvation.
Taken from composite data from 5 studies, assembled by Elia, 1991.

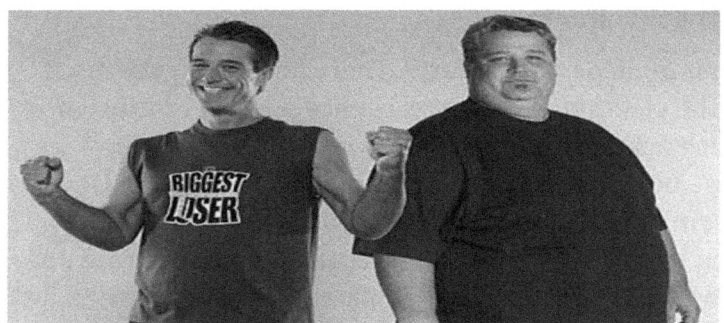

Illustration 1: Danny Cahill Regained the weight he lost on a calorie restriction high exercise diet

The biggest Loser TV show shows us why conventional diets don't lead to long term weight loss for most people – the metabolic damage stays with them and that makes it ever harder to lose weight. Studies showed that people who did the show which involved intensive exercise and minimal calories but still eating every day – their metabolism never recovered. That doesn't happen with water fasting. It's more extreme so you would think water fasting would produce more damage. But actually its a natural function – our bodies have a special mode it goes into with a water fast.

That's why it's so important not to eat anything at all in this special mode – not one bite! This is a protective and healing mode that came from us living through winters. The body knows how to do it and switch to fat burning and running off ketones rather than carbohydrates. So the body is actually still "eating" full meals every day, it's just doing it from your own fat. It takes a few days to get into this mode unless you are already on a strict keto diet.

Going on a keto diet first then doing a water fast will be easier because the body is already in a burn fat mode. If you aren't it's just a few days for the body to shift into it, but they can be crappy hungry days on the water fast. Which is why one day fasts don't do so much (unless you are deep in a keto diet and producing ketones).

The Re-Feeding Collapse Danger

Why not 30 days fast? There have been issue with refeeding. Mainly with malnourished people, where your body does a strange phosphate loss and people can die. Typically if it happens you need to get to the hospital immediately and they will intravenous give you phosphorous. This is one reason for adding in the bone broth towards the end of the fast and building up your phosphorous and salts. It does add a 50 calorie per glass hit, so it can stop some of the good things happening. But for safety, it's important to rebuild before you finish your fast.

Again, this re-feeding syndrome is quite rare, but you should know about it for your own safety. Be careful when you break your fast.

Why not every other day fasting?

There are a few reasons why every other day fasting wont be nearly as effective. The first problem is you'll be hungry like a demon. Your hunger doesn't turn off in a fast until day five. They the rest of the days are pretty much home free. So it can be just so difficult to do this every other day protocol.... until you are a lot healthier and stronger. But there are other reasons as well.

I'll go into this a bit later, but basically your liver and pancreas have become stuffed with fat. This is a lot of the reason why you are diabetic. If this gets too extreme you can actually kill off all the beta cells on your pancreas and become a type 1 diabetic. Studies which looked at the liver and hepatic fat found that after two weeks of fasting EIGHTY PERCENT of the liver fat was flushed away. EIGHTY PERCENT IN TWO WEEKS. Let's take a look at the liver and see this for ourselves.

Hepatic Fat

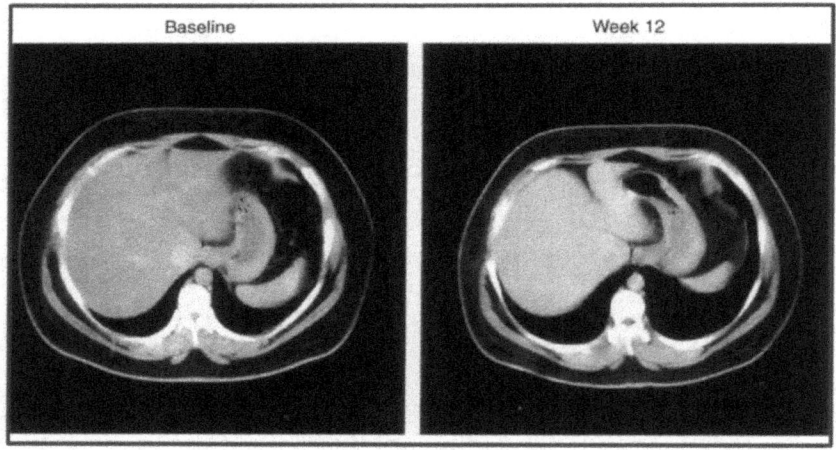

Mean loss of liver volume 28.7%
80% by first 2 weeks

Preoperative weight loss with a very-low-energy diet Am J Cli Nutr 2006;84:304-311

So if you don't fast for two or three weeks, this won't happen. And getting that liver to flush out its fat is a huge key to getting back to health. Don't think of yourself as diabetic, think of yourself as having fatty liver and fatty pancreas. You have to get the fat out. And that takes time. So if 80 percent flushes in two weeks, in ten days it should make a fair comeback. And while there's less research on the pancreas, we can expect similar things to happen. A study in mice found beta cell (the thingies that make insulin) regeneration from fasting. Not confirmed in humans, but likely.

So the fat basically flushes out of your body this way. First from your organs like your liver and pancreas. That's great news because it means you don't have to get skinny before you can recover! Next the interstitial fats that belly tube flush out. And finally fat everywhere. Also glucose begins to burn off. I thought that glucose would be gone in a day but no – see calculating your magic day. It was amazing to see HOW MUCH GLUCOSE my body was full of and how long it took to get burned off.

Now one more point of flushing out liver fat. Apparently so much fat flushes out that it carries ALT with it, which is a standard metabolic test marker for liver malfunction. If your ALT was normal before the fast but high after, then this might be what is happening, it's benign and should clear up in 16 weeks (see the section on Research to read the study). What this means is that if your doctor freaks out, show them the study and say "It's because I water fasted causing fat to flush from the liver – a good thing!"

So on the longer fast, by about day five hunger is just flat gone. And a few days after that energy goes up. Once in that mode, the main issues are headaches (which treat easily with aspririn or Excedrin liquid gels for a bad one), bad breath (get the peppermint spray), and a bit of weakness. Well you are fasting you aren't supposed to be chopping wood for gods sake! So really you could just continue, but remember, once Hunger returns you should break the fast. Your body is telling you it's time.

If you experience any abdominal pain even slight pain, that's another sign to break the fast, although some rumbling is normal. If you experience sharp pains up toward your right rib where your gallbladder is, that's an emergency sign to get to a doctor asap (see chapter on gallstones). Because of some of the rare bad things that happen on people doing 30 or 100 day water fasts, I do like to keep it to 10 or 14 days, and just fast several times. I am not certain, but I would guess there's much lower incidence of problems with the shorter fast. Another issue is that for the longer fasts, you really want to be monitored which means being inpatient at a clinic and that can get expensive.

The Four Bags of Fat and How We Get Diabetes

It's taken ten to twenty years for you to get diabetic and it's been fairly hidden the whole time. Every year things getting worse and worse but without much outside evidence to show for it except weight gain. To understand how this happens I want to talk about your four bags of fat.

The first bag of fat is your organs – of specific importance your liver and pancreas. Slowly year after year of eating EITHER too many carbohydrates OR of not having long enough down periods between eating (what happened to me, I'd eat late into the night) your body gets stuck needing to put the extra stuff which regardless if its fats or carbs it converts to fat. And slowly year after year your liver and pancreas start to fill up. It's called non-alcoholic fatty liver disease and it's becoming very common. I don't think diabetes is possible without it. Now your organs are pretty tough. It might take 20 years to stuff so much fat in that they begin failing. Then when they flip over to failure BANG blood sugars go up and you are diabetic.

The second bag of fat is interstitial abdominal fat. Some of this is brown adipose tissue. The great thing about brown adipose tissue is if you eat a big meal, it can just blast it off you by transforming it to heat. As a person without a thyroid, I couldn't do this. Another reason I got so sick. But regular people do. Which is why you see people like Mark Weins (the world food reviewer on youtube) eat five thousand calories a day and stay stick thin. But there's another horrible case where bag 2 gets screwed up. Once you start being diabetic and your insulin rises to try to cram fat into cells already full (like a bicycle pump putting more and more air into a tire) well that insulin does something terrible to bag 2. Research shows that it shuts down this burn off as heat wasting function and switches everything over to put more fat on mode. So once you get even just a teensy tiny bit diabetic, you're doomed.

The third bag of fat is the fat that's in all our muscles and tissues generally. Places where the insulin has stuffed it.

The fourth bag of fat is the fat that's the jiggly fat we see on fat people. What's interesting is genetically some fat people never direct fat into bag 1 – the organs, and go straight to bag four. And they get huge. But they never get diabetes. This is the "my 600 pound life" people. Eventually their hearts fail unable to keep up with the huge bodies.

The reason understanding the four bags of fat is important is that you have to realize you put the fat on in bag 1, then bag 2, then bag 3, then bag 4. When your fat comes off, it will come off In the same order. So don't pull on your love handle and feel disappointed. There's a ton of good things happening inside! You just can't see it. Eventually bags 1-3 will empty out and then the jiggly fats will begin going away. Now of course it's not as strict as all that, but you can think about it that way.

Now I have a friend and he is one of those weird genetic anomalies where he didn't really use bag 1 and get diabetes. Instead he just kept blasting out bag 4 fat and getting bigger and bigger. When you've met one of these types of people they are very quick to see. They have good energy, no diabetes, just their body kept growing and growing so they are MASSIVE. This is most likely NOT YOU. They would also benefit from water fasting, but a much longer medically supervised in hospital fast until the weight is off. Instead our medical system takes these people and cuts their stomachs out, there's a huge risk of death from anesthesia and complications. Our medical system is horrific and stupid. So if you know someone like this and they are considering or being pressured into the stomach surgery, please give them this book or tell them about water fasting. Being on such a long fast, they will need nutritional supplements beyond bone broth.

The doctors are quite mad and stuffed with bad research telling them to chop out stomachs. Here is one example "For unknown reasons, sudden or quick weight loss achieved through dietary modification may lead to the progression of liver failure in some NAFLD patients [32]. On the other hand, weight reduction through surgical methods, even with quick weight-loss after surgery, has been successful in reducing disease progression" - Is there any Consensus as to what Diet or lifestyle Approach Is the Right one for NAFID Patients? Carmine Finelli1 , Giovanni Tarantino1,2 1) Center of Obesity and Eating Disorder, Stella Maris Mediterraneum Foundation, Chiaromonte, Potenza; 2) Department of Clinical and Experimental Medicine, Federico II University Medical School of Naples, Naples, Italy

NOTE: they did not include fasting in their study.

This of course, totally ignores the reversal of NAFLD through fasting. And as we have seen, these exercise a lot restrict calories that the doctors put sick patients on are dangerous. I think the reason for this is you are still forcing the fatty liver to work 100% through this crazy period. With the water fasting, instead it's a period of rest for the organ, rest and regeneration.

I never can figure out why they cut out peoples stomachs at all other than they are surgeons and that's how they get paid, isn't it so much safer just to wire these peoples jaws shut? Probably psychologically they can't handle the thought of not being able to eat and chew food at all. Total lack of will power. I had jaw surgery for my bite and couldn't eat anything for eight weeks. It's totally possible!

Calculating your "Magic Day"

I began my fast with a blood glucose of 340. On day six I tested it again. 186. What the HECK! Yep it's true, your body is so stuffed with glucose that it takes a while to get it down. In my case I calculated a rate of about 25 points a day. So that meant I would have to wait until day 10 for my "magic day".

Let's say your fasting glucose is 200. so to get down to 100 you need to drop 100 points. That should be about four or five days of fasting.

One reason to calculate your magic day is that it gives you an early point to work towards and look forward to in your fast which can otherwise be a bit rough at the beginning.

Ok why is it a magic day? Because once you get your blood sugar under 100 all that thirst and peeing and drinking STOPS. It's over. Hopefully forever. Oh my god. Bliss. Also that dizziness and weakness, also should be a lot better. So calculate your magic day. If you were totally F-ed like me it might take ten days. But it will happen. So this is one reason why its good to keep checking your blood sugar. As you see it drop every day it will motivate you to stay on the fast. And seeing the pounds fly off on the scale (usually between 0.8 and 1.2 pounds a day).

How NOT to fast

So before I began my fast I watched a LOT of youtube videos on fasting. A lot! And on diabetes theory, low carb diets, everything. For like two years. Seriously a lot!

So I came across one video and I won't describe it too much in detail but basically the guy fasted by only drinking distilled water. Whaaaaaa???? So he was getting no minerals. That's life threatening! Don't ever do that! And nothing else. Then he described his fast as going to school and studying for several hours then hitting the gym for a few hours. Then he smiles and says he lost two pounds a day.

This is not how to fast. First thing to remember is think of yourself as a big bear. We were designed for periods of no food. The bear climbs into his cave and rests through winter. Interestingly, Chimps being tropical with no winters cannot fast. Fast a chimp and they quickly die. Fast a human and we switch over to fat burning and a ketone metabolism within five days.

So I think its critical that you plan to be in bed for much of your fast. No cleaning. No exercise. Rest. Rest a lot. Only when your energy levels return SO HIGH that you CAN'T STAND to stay in bed should you get up. I would say that regardless of how you feel you should plan on just being in bed for the first two weeks regardless. The protocol of healing and regeneration REQUIRES THE REST.

Now can you work? I did. I didn't have much of a problem working. But I did it from my bed. And I took breaks and rested several times. So before you start your fast if you go to an office to work, make arrangements to work from home for the month. It's medical if they balk get a doctors not. This is about SAVING YOUR LIFE. If they still say no FK em.

This fast is about SAVING YOUR LIFE. And based on two years of research it's the only way. This is serious shit. Do not ever take it lightly.

So remember, one time only, you are going to become a bear and rest and "hibernate". And your body is going to recognize what's going on and do amazing things.

Are you a mom who has kids and makes all the meals. Maybe you need to do your fast away from home in a fasting center. And make plans for the family to have another caretaker during your fast. Because you simply cannot get in the long rests and low activity you need to do during the fast if you are being a provider to others.

Rest.   Rest.   Stay in bed as much as you can possibly stand it. Take it slow and easy. This is so important I cannot over emphasize it.   The body wants to go into a bear-hibernate mode. If you are doing jumping jacks or making dinner for four, your body is going to get confused as to what is going on and you won't get the critical regeneration cycle.

One amazing thing that happens is autophagy which means killing off unneeded cells and clearing out the cobwebs and junk. This is a critical path for people who might be fighting cancer.

And it DOES NOT HAPPEN on short fasts. So this fast is fixing many many things. All those albumin molecules which collect in the brain and cause alzheimers – research is coming out showing fasting can help.

So again, do not go to the gym, don't go to the office. Close the blinds, set up your bed as a nice comfy place, watch some movies on your computer, and rest and sleep when your body tells you to. And dear god don't drink distilled water!

Since you are drinking ONLY water (and a broth I will tell you about shortly) what water should you drink. All I can say is avoid those gallon jugs of water. They have bleach. What ever water quenches your thirst. If that's a non sparkling non mineral water, then keep that whatever it is for your main water supply but fine some mineral water to add to that so you are getting some minerals in.

NO ARTIFICIAL SWEETNERS. NONE. No sorbitol, xylitol, truvia, NOTHING. And it goes without saying NOTHING with SUGAR.

The Danger of Gall Stones

One of the possibilities which might occur, although rare, is gallstones. The reason is that you are flushing a lot of fat from the liver into the gallbladder. The gallbladder gets somewhat overloaded and also the fats being flushed go along with a lot of other built up ick from the liver. What can happen is a small gall stone can block the outgoing bile duct from the gallbladder. This results in very sharp abdominal pain. So if you suddenly feel a terrible pain in your abdomen, get to a doctor quick. Normally these can be treated but in worst case surgery to remove the entire gallbladder is performed. This is almost unheard of on a 10 day fast. But just know the association is there.

Tummy Massages

A couple of times a day, relax, lay flat on your back, and using your palms gently massage your abdomen Especially if you find hard spots or sore spots. Your intestines are in a bit of a state of shock and digestion has shut down. Massaging your abdomen can help thing s feel better. Just push in long strokes from top to bottom, from side to side. Turn on your left side and your abdomen will shift. Massage again. Turn on your right side and again massage. I found these abdomen massages helpful. Since you are resting and aren't so busy, it's another thing to do to pass the time.

Setting Up For Your Fast – Secret Tricks and Tips and Things to Get

Ugh well when I started my fast I didn't have time to get ready at all. But slowly I realized there's a lot of things I needed. So lets go over your shopping list.

Obviously you should have all your prescriptions. But remember since you aren't eating ANYTHING then you won't need diabetes medications (check with your doctor of course). But make sure you are covered for your 30 day fast period.

Next is water. I kept driving to the store for water. Big mistake. Eventually I bought it in more and bigger quantities – clearing out the stores stock! So basically I'd recommend skipping this you don't want to have to get up and drive and shop. Get all your water up front. If you are satiated with just your tap water, find a good mineral water you like to supplement. Because you will need minerals. If your already diabetic peeing you already know about higher water needs.

Next is aspirin. Just regular 325 gram aspirin tablets. Four the first five days of the fast take two every morning. Because headaches is one of the things that happen in the adjustment period. And they can be bad. For something faster and strong also pick up some liquid Excedrin gel caps. Those work really well. Will you for sure get headaches? Most likely you will. But this will help.

Burts Bees Lip Balm. I found my lips really dried out. But this has a secondary function more than just your lips. When you fast your body will push out all kinds of horrors. From everywhere. From your skin, from sweats, from your breath, and from your pee. And it will all stink like a turd. A horrible turd. The burts bees has peppermint oil. So rather than smelling stinky breath, it will cover it up a bit. Which leads us to....

Get a KETO Breath meter. This is more useful for after the fast to make sure your keto eating is working, but its great to see your body is DEEP in keto during the fast. Your numbers during the fast will be quadruple what they will be when eating keto. It's encouraging to see a sign that things are really happening. This is OPTIONAL. Yes there are keto pee strips but ... ick.

Peppermint breath spray. The important thing is to make SURE it is zero calorie and doesn't have ANY of the fake sweeteners. Xylitol, Sorbitol, Truvia. NO way. Pay a bit more and get a good one. This will save you from smelling your stinky breath. And along that line there is also....

Infowars Blue Flouride Free Toothpaste. You get it from Infowars.com's store.   It's fluoride free and has iodine, silver, and tons of peppermint. Sadly even with this strong stuff you'll still smell stinky breath. But well .. it helps.

Teas. One tea to get is ginger tea. That's for when your tummy is rumbling. Green tea. And maybe an occasional tea that has a bit of caffeine, but don't guzzle on it. I got English breakfast tea, but I never really got a craving for it. So get the ginger tea, and make sure you have a selection of teas. In the first few days of your fast when your tummy is gurgling and complaining, hit it with a nice hot ginger tea. It will really help.

What about Bullion cubes? NO! They are too artificial and have too much salt. NOT ALLOWED. But this is where the broth comes in.

Ok finally is vegetables for broth. Wait this is a water fast! What the heck! This is a zero calorie broth or very close to zero. And its basically taken when you feel you need it. Essentially about every other day. The broth is super simple. Just three things. Celery, baby carrots, and organic red pepper. Get a good amount of each and 2 large red peppers. That will cover two broth makings. Then have way through get fresh veggies and do again. The celery has a lot of minerals and the veggies help to get a bit of nutrition into you. To make the broth I used my instapot. Put the strainer in first then several bunches of celery (whole) half the bag of carrots, and 1 pepper just broken a bit into pieces. Pressure cooked it for 30 minutes and it was done. When it cooled a bit put the veggies down the garbage disposal. Easy peasy. If you don't have a pressure cooker you can use a crock pot for a few hours on high, or just in a large pot boiling. I would say its a bit more than a quart of water. You don't want TOO much water as you want a strong broth.

Once its ready put just enough salt in that it tastes neutral but good. Do not put in salt to make it taste salty. That little bit of salt will really help you during the fast. You'll know when you need it because you'll head for the broth. Warm it up good and hot. It's really a fast saver and will get you through when you think you cant make it. One big coffee mug full is plenty. Just once a day max. I found I only wanted it like every other day.

Fasting Failure... What NOT to Do!

You really have to commit to the rest required for the fast. You have to tone things down and rest in bed. The biggest thing that will cause you to fail on your fast is to try to do too much. Failure to properly rest a lot will ruin your fast. Other things that can ruin your fasts is to continue to pound yourself with caffeine, diet drinks, etc. It's best to break your addictions to these BEFORE the fast.

Don't leave yourself a lot of house chores to do before the fast and don't do any of that during the fast. Remember it's about REST. You are a big grizzly bear climbing into your comfortable cave for a long winters rest!

Last Day of Fast Decisions

This chapter has some breaking the fast info BUT read "BREAKING THE FAST" chapter below its even more important even if the information is overlapping.

It's day 10 of your fast. And you feel great. Can you extend the fast to 15 days? Yes you can. The key question is DO YOU FEEL HUNGRY? When I reached day 10 I felt hunger creeping in. And I felt a soreness in part of my abdomen Both signs to break the fast.

But if you just feel no hunger, reasonable energy (obviously you might not feel full energy on a fast) then yes you can continue to 15 days with more benefit. People routinely under medical programs do a 30 day fast (I don't recommend due to the rare chance of the refeeding issue see that chapter). So 15 days is not really that long for a fast. Remember the longest recorded fast is 385 days. Some overweight people, feeling no hunger just keep fasting until all the weight is off.

But that is not the strategy I recommend. We are fasting to get the liver and pancreas de-fatted. Not to get the weight off. And you do that to 80% in 14 days. It's probably 65 or 70% in 10.

OK you've decided to break your fast. You should have your break your fast food ready. I recommend berries – strawberries, blueberries, blackberries, olliolaberies – and home made sugar free whipped cream from heavy cream and vanilla extract.

Remember on the day you are breaking your fast you DO NOT EAT FULL MEALS. This is your first day back to eating. What did I do? About 6 large organic strawberries with copious amounts of whipped cream, and I ate that twice, once in late morning, and once around 6pm. Remember you aren't hungry yet, so it's not like you have to gorge!

Then next 3-4 days you will be in "sensitive" mode. No steaks! No ground beef. Bacon in small amounts seems to be ok as it crumbles quite tiny, scrambled eggs with whipped cream never causes tummy pains. Continue with berries and cream. Fresh mozzarella balls (soft!). I like my jars of artichoke hearts in oil eaten with a skewer. Olives. But don't go for the big meals and steaks just yet. After another day try a soft fish like cod. The first few times you eat you will MOST LIKELY experience tummy pains and need to rest. Your system is re-adjusting it's nothing to get overly concerned about. Eat small, wait and see how your tummy is doing. After a few days of this try a bit more of a challenging food. Finally after 3 days you should be ready for steak – but chew well.

Sensitivities post fast: You WILL be overly sensitive to SALT and SUGAR. Of course you aren't putting sugar in any food but if you were to go out to eat and they had put sugar in you would immediately sense it (and hopefully go YUK!). Put in only the tiniest pinches of salt, nothing like the amounts you used before.

Stage 2: Post Fast Strategy

It's hard to predict what your post fast level of recovery will be. Certainly one hopes that things will be much improved, but that doesn't mean you can go gobble loaves of bread and bagels and be fine right after the fast. If you still aren't at goal weight (and that's likely because in a thirty day fast you aren't going to lose more than 35 pounds) then you still most likely will need to avoid carbs.

So now you are at stage 2. And in this stage you are going to be on a very low carb High Healthy Fats diet. Not forever. Once you are fully trim you will be able to add back some carbs.

Watch Dr. Nina Teicholz videos on the importance of Meat and Fat in our diets and the dangers of processed oils. And dig up some KETO meal guides. Remember KETO means NOT JUST GORGING ON MEAT in fact your meat portion per day is actually fairly small. And don't gorge on cheese and nuts either. A good KETO meal plan has non starchy vegetables, some meat and eggs and dairy, and mostly fat. That fat should come from a natural source – Lard, Suet, Butter, Tallow. You can have a bit of olive oil on salad but never cook with olive oil. When I make bacon I save the fat in the refrigerator then I use that on salads, on vegetables, it's a flavorful way to add extra fat to a meal.

When I make eggs I add whole cream. Another trick to boost fat! When I snack I have a few berries with whipping cream (no sugar and home made). YUM! Yes you can eat a few macadamia nuts (the best nut) each day, but not a pound of them! I like to go out for Thai Thom Ka Goog (coconut milk spicy soup with shrimp) but you must tell them NO SUGAR. In fact eating out is almost impossible beyond getting a steak. Avoid fast food places they doctor and put crap stuff in EVERYTHING and never ever eat fast food french fries cooked in destroyed vegetable oil. Yah NO vegetable oil for you again EVER. NEVER. That's Wesson, Rapeseed, Sunflower, Corn, Canola, Crisco, etc. All will destroy your organs.

I love croissants. So one thing I have is a Once a Month cheat. Its good to see how much you are recovered and how you will handle some carbohydrates so it's a good test as well! But it can't be a full plate of spaghetti. More like one fork full. Or maybe a bit of cake. Then test your glucose 2 hours later. If it's in normal range – under 140 - then congrats you have restored Beta cell and insulin function and lesser insulin resistance! Next month try a bit more carbs and see what happens. But it's unlikely that you should return breads and carbs to your daily eating, it just might make you sick again and who wants that after going through so much to get better!

Breaking Your Fast – VERY IMPORTANT TO READ THIS !!!

When you end your fast you DO NOT just begin eating regular meals again. NO!

Instead you need to very gradually introduce SOFT foods and in small amounts. For example I am breaking my fast with two strawberries very well chewed with whipped cream. Other people like berries and yogurt. DO NOT break your fast by drinking Orange Juice or other fruit juices. That is forbidden on keto diet anyways but it would immediately stress your insulin system with a huge glucose load. Break your fast with a KETO high fat portion of maybe 200 calories. Do not break your fast with MEAT or with GRAINS. NO TOAST OR BREAD. You could break your fast with some cooked mushy pumpkin. Or other non starchy vegetable. Again, just a few tablespoons. Then four hours later another "meal" of 200 calories. You are seeing how your stomach responds. You hopefully will not get cramps and pain if you follow this advice. If you do NOT follow this advice you WILL get terribly painful digestion pain for hours. FOLLOW THIS ADVICE. Don't break your fast with applesauce or other forms of a pure fruit. Even the sugar free will be too glucose based. Do not break your fast with NUTS. You could break your fast with some full fat cottage cheese. But don't break your fast with regular cheese. Most non starchy vegetables could be used to break the fast provided you have added butter for a fat source. Mashed cauliflower with butter and a bit of water to make it very thin almost like a soup. For me, a few berries and whipped cream is a good way to do it. Home made whipped cream – just cream and vanilla flavoring extract. NO SUGAR!

There is a product called Yakult which is a kefir. I don't recommend it. It's fat free and has artificial sugar. You could use a full fat greek yogurt that's sugar free like Fage along with fruit to break your fast but I find it a bit too thick so I prefer just to make my own whipped cream.

So when you break the fast, don't do it in the morning. Try to wait to 11am or noon. Then give it four hours. See how the stomach responds. It might be a bit gurgly but that's ok. As long as you don't get pain and cramps. If you do get a bit of a painful reaction, when you next have your mini portion add some water and make sure its well mashed up or chewed even longer. After the second meal things should start feeling a bit more normal.

Four hours later (7pm) eat for the THIRD TIME, again just a 200 calorie mini snack of the same thing you had at 11am and 3pm. You have now had 600 calories and you digestive system knows its back on food. So does your brain. Your body knows your water fast is over. Tomorrow, you can have breakfast.

The Next Day:

OK ready for the first REAL MEAL. I'm having eggs with cream and bacon. The eggs cooked in two pats of butter. Be sure to chew EXTRA LONG so everything is very well broken up. You want the less stress on your stomach as possible. If you make it through breakfast, you can have a salad for lunch and get some veggies in. I really recommend pastured eggs for your first real meal. they have so many key nutrients that will re-feed you. Your body will suck it up.

What's it's like to fast – My Journal

Day 1:

Holy crap I'm dying. I'm really going to do this. I'm pretty scared
but determined. Once you get THAT sick this is kind of like take
your medicine. You worked too hard and ignored your health for
too long. But I take solace in knowing this is a ONE TIME THING.
That really helped mentally. I just have to get through it. Can I.
The American diabetes association says I don't have the will
power. Fk them. I do.

As I said, with your liver and pancreas full of fat, theirs no
winning. That's why fasting – longer term fasting of ten days or
more is the better solution. I know Dr. Fung gets recoveries with
fasts of just 8 days but stronger patients go fast as long as they
feel good. Other patients don't do a longer term fast and get
there with KETO and some other day fasting. Some people can
even get the fat out with just high exercise but as we've
discussed with the "biggest loser" tv show, while this may lead
to wellness, it also destroys your basal metabolic rate, even for
years and years. So it's not worth doing. The best approach is
fast for 10 days, then after that hurdle go to KETO eating and do
that for a while, and then if you need it you can try for the 14
day water fast to get more weight off and more fat out of the
liver. Plus, It's just sooo much easier to get on a fast and stay on
it than to go on off on off. Getting through that first four day is
the tough part, so if you do shorter fasts, your in hell almost all
the fast. With what i'm doing now, it's just four days of meh..
not great not the worst thing in the world. It's a mental game,
you against your body screams Carbs... Bagels... Pancakes... feed
me. And you must win.

Symptoms. Headache is starting. Stomach is kinda gurgly and painful. It wants it's food. It isn't getting it. Took my aspirin and head is a bit better. Just rested in bed all day. I know that the first four days are harder then it gets better. It's just a wait it out thing. Rest. Watch videos on fasting. Watch Jason Fung's video. He's a bit of a weasel not telling you his exact protocol ;*> But I still love him. Because he's the first doctor saving people from diabetes.

Day 2:

Hunger is definitely worse. I drink my ginger tea. Later I drink my broth. Holy shit that helped. That nice warm broth. Calmed the tummy right down. Rest and rest and more rest. More headaches. More aspirin. I'm not super hungry. It's a weird feeling. More like unsettled. Just bide my time and get through.

Day 3:

It's day Three! I'm pretty happy that I'm sticking with it. I had to get out and get more water at the store. I stopped by the evil clinic that never gave me my meds and told them I was doing better but I needed my friggin meds (they never did give them to me). I do some stuff for work and then I realize I have to clean up a bit. Big mistake I'm too weak to do it. I barely grab a bag upstairs to throw out old bottles. I'm fine laying, but every time I get up its like I've got 120 seconds before I have to scramble back in bed and rest. Just dizzy weak. Ugh. Breath smells like a rat died in there. Horrible. But I know I'm almost through the tough part. So I focus on bed rest. I'm almost over the tough part.

Day 4:

It's day four. I should be past the hard part but I'm not. I'm still is crappy hell mode. I try to drink a lot I'm still frequently peeing but I notice its less frequent and more pee is coming out. That huge urgency to pee has diminished. Rat breath continues. But I've got my burts bees now and that helps a bit. I brush my teeth but it provides minimal relief.

Day 5: Breakthrough

I wake up and suddenly I feel a lot different. I'm not quite up to power by any means. I know instantly I've broken into ketosis. Hunger is gone. Stomach rumbles are gone. I weigh in. lost six pounds. Good. Seeing the weight come off on the scale really helps motivate you to continue. By ten days my weight will be lower than its been in a decade. I can't wait to get my weight down. Yes that sounds ridiculous but... considering I started at very obese it's an almost impossible mountain. I calculate that by then end of the fast if I'm lucky I should just barely crack 15 pounds lost. I know I didn't have ANY diabetic symptoms when I was eighty pounds lighter. So I should be very close to healed. I'll have to do the LCHF and alternate day fasting when I finish to do the more gradual healing and weight loss. But hopefully with the liver and pancreas flushed out the function will come back. No idea if it will or wont. There's just no way of knowing its just a hope. I've got some big projects to finish up for work so I do that. Then I watch a will Farrell movie that makes me cry. I go to bed at 10:30. I notice I'm sleeping a lot less.

Day 6:

I ordered a different glucose test kit that's a lot more advanced. Like it has date and time, memory, and can calculate averages. It even has a data port to upload to your notebook. But I still can't stick myself. But today they do that at the grocery. I've finally gotten my thyroid prescription from the other doctor not the shit place so I'm off to pick that up. Driving was fine but when it came to standing... wuf. I'm still sick. It's not the fast its the diabetes. Just cant stand but I have to to get everything. The glucose test nurse was so sweet. She was very efficient but I was shocked to see that even six days of no food my glucose was only down to 186 (see the magic number). Grrr. Jesus I must have been stuffed to the gills with glucose. I calculate that it's going to be day TEN before its normal. GRRR. I'm impatient. By the time I get my water and hit checkout I'm woozy. I barely get home, get the water in the fridge up the stairs and into bed. I'm visibly gasping as I finally flop over. God its good to be back to rest. This is why I Do NOT recommend going out shopping during the fast. Stay in bed! Stay in BED.

Day 7:

Today again no hunger. Its nice. What a time saver. So much time going into cooking, eating, cleaning up, its practically half your life. You don't know that until you stop eating. I've woken up feeling a lot more energy but I'm still having trouble standing. I realize I was really seriously close to full diabetic ketoacidosis. Maybe death. I call my sister and tell her whats going on. I try to write a small will to make sure she'll get stuff if I croak. Ya never know. I think that thought that knowing I had reached a really serious level of sickness is making me take this water fast VERY seriously. And of course I want to be better. Weight is down nine pounds and all I can think of is getting below the next goal. Weight loss seems to slow but I know it can't. I should hit my magic number and get there in just three days. I can't wait!

Standing up is a little better than before. But the best thing is my diabetic numb feet seem to be better. I've been taking PQQ which helps a lot with nerves. But the lower glucose and the weight loss I duno its like I can walk again. I tell myself I can't be having big effects like that this quickly. I realize too my horror my broth recipe has produced too stinky broth because I put in parsley and mushrooms. So I have to redo it. All I need is a red pepper. So I'll get that my next trip to the grocery. Having a lighter non stinky broth will really help. And you can sorta tell you need that salt from the broth every couple days. I'm drinking my Mineraga which is non mineral carbonated water, and its not great. The Topo chico is much better but a pain in the small bottles. Bottles are everywhere. I go downstairs and grab a grocery bag and bring it up. Again totally wheezed out from that small effort. I've been giving myself one small task a day to do. Got my Burts bees lip balm yay. Thank you amazon. It helps a bit with the dead turd in my mouth. And I've ordered peppermint spray. Omg that will be amazing. You wont have to suffer like me, I've gathered all these things into the book!

Day 8:

Today was a weird day. I got up and scaled. Down 11 pounds. Wow, that sticky weight that didn't seem to drop has now dropped. So that is a weight I haven't seen in a very long time and it's sorta my first goal. I worked today. I also noticed that my standing dizziness and weakness is getting better as if I'm slowly getting more endurance again. But then in the afternoon I had this not exactly hunger, just a huge urge to want to eat again and it was mainly mental. I told myself I need to shorten the fast I cant possibly make 30 days. But then after drinking a good bit as they day got to 7pm I realized I was feeling a lot better. Close to normal. I'm one day from sticking myself. So I dragged out this Owell kit I ordered from amazon. The reason I got a new glucose test kit is like a dope I left a test strip in my old unit and it burned out the battery. I tried to open the battery compartment and couldn't figure it out. So screw it it's only 24 bucks. The thing is, I didn't test myself with the old unit because the needle pen had this really hard button. I just couldn't push it hard enough. Well the new stuff has a much nicer unit with dates, times, memories, data logs, etc. But even the needle pen was a lot better. Very easy to adjust down to wimp level stick and a softer button. Nice. Also it says I can stick the palm of my hand not my finger tips as long as I'm fasting. Which of course I am. So tomorrow I will try to do the blood stick and see hopefully a glucose under 100.

Day 9:

Last night I felt clear. I think it was hitting my normal blood sugar for the first time. I'll check it today. My weight is down 13 pounds lost in 8-9 days. So I am tracking much above one pound a day. I think that's normal for fatter people but to be honest I wasn't that optimistic. I hope I get near 20 pounds lost by the time I end the fast on day 15. I won't quite hit my goal of being in down 30 pounds but I should get close!

It's really coming down fast now. And my stomach is almost... almost back to near flat. Therese still a bit of blubber on one side. But it's getting close. That means I've switches to what I call BAG 2 of fat – interstitial belly. Which hopefully means that the organs are all mostly cleared out.

I'm a bit worried I will still be in a state of near total pancreas dysfunction when I exit my fast. This isn't enough time for it to recover. But on the near zero carb eating you still have protein which uses insulin so I have to be very careful to watch things as I begin eating. My sugars could just go straight up, in which case I'll have to fast for a day and then keep trying. From the doctors lectures I've seen, it's three months to some recovery of beta cells, but, of course you might not get any if you are too damaged. I believe in the body's power to heal itself so I'm trying to be optimistic. There's very little data on people who do a longer fast and then how their pancreas recovers. Theres much more on the liver. And from what I've seen, NAFL can totally recover in just a bit over two weeks of fasting. I'm nervous but hopeful.

Today I have to do a blood test. I'll do it later as I perk up in the afternoon. Just took my thyroid meds. My car battery died so I got grocery store delivery. 20 20oz bottles of topo chico and 8 cartons of pre made bone broth. I looked at their recipe and it's exactly what the recipe is on line so... how bad can premade be? Theres a more expensive one which is grass fed which I found on amazon. So I blew 20 bucks on just 3 of them, but one is chicken mushroom which sounds nice. So starting today I'll add 8oz of bone broth and then tomorrow 16oz from then to the end of the fast. That should ensure I don't have mineral issues. The downside? Its 50 calories a cup so it might stop autophagy and other good things. But on the other hand it's so minimal amount of calories I think it will be ok. Dr. Fung uses bone broth and he gets recoveries so I should be ok. I trust in Dr. Fung! But I do think this is another case where you can prepare for your fast (I was in emergency mode so I couldn't) and pre-make it fresh and it will be much better. I don't care so much about taste. Just the nutrients. (opens and drinks the pre-made bone broth) ... Uhm I take it back I do care about the taste. The pre made stuff is disgusting. Definitely make your own bone broth. Freeze half of it for fresh stuff in week 2.

My trying to test my blood didn't go well. I tried to get blood from my palm. 4 painful sticks later – no blood. Ouch. OK I'll do the finger. Set up the test strip in the machine. Pushed the button on the pen with it against my finger. OUCH! OK theirs blood. Put the blood on the test strip. Machine flashes "G-1" bad test strip. FUCK. Take out a new test strip. Put in machine. Squeeze finger. No more blood. F-k it. F-k this. I ordered a KETO breath meter. All I have to do is blow in. If I'm in ketosis I can't have high glucose. Right? Maybe I'll just do that. I know I have to get a glucose level but I feel great. Most of the sick is gone. Energy isn't perfect but I can now finally stand and do simple things like go down the stairs and grab water and climb the stairs back up all without getting too dizzy. Its progress. Told a nice woman at work I was on day 9 of fasting and she freaked. EAT she screamed. She harped on that I needed a candy bar or something for a while. I promised I would eat in a couple days. Six days to be exact but I didn't tell her that part. I am starting to dream about a keto meal of eggs and bacon in butter with cream. Enough to break the fast early. But I'll stick it out.

(night time)

I've noticed a painful area in my lower left abdomen. Like its hard. It seems too low to be the gallbladder which is up higher in the abdomen. Still I take caution and see it as a warning sign that I should probably break the fast. The other is I got hungry. When hunger returns, regardless of the day, break your fast. It's not worth complications. So please remember that. When hunger returns, regardless of when, break your fast (with the break fast protocol).

Day 10:

OK I've made it. Sure it's not the LONGEST FAST but it is dramatic nonetheless. I weighed in at 16 pounds lost in ten days. And since today is technically by calorie intake a fast day (just not a complete water fast day) a bit more weight will come off. Of course after eating a few pounds will go back on right away from having stuff in your digestive tract again. But it feels like an accomplishment. My stomach is much closer to flat than before. My mobility and walking around is hugely different. It's like I went from a Hippo to Light on my feet. Yes 16 pounds makes that much of a difference. From my start, I've now dropped 50 pounds. And now I'll go onto keto diet so weight will continue to come off. Please remember when you break your fast this day you eat VERY LIGHT. No real eating until the NEXT DAY. I Am having two strawberries with whipped cream in the morning, then again in the afternoon. That's it. So this day is not a regular eating day. You have to let your body learn to recognize food again. It's frustrating not to jump into eggs and bacon but ... very very important.

I went from very sickly to feeling pretty good. Energy levels have gone up every single day. I think that's a sign that even without food my liver is recovering. Sure it would be good to go another week without food and get that 80 % fat flush in the liver, but you know what, from a difficulty level I think you can get 90% of the benefit with half the effort on the 10 day fast. The advantage of these longer term fasts is you both get that organ fat flush as well as giving your digestive and insulin systems a needed break. The poor pancreas has been over pumping insulin for years. I pray I have some insulin recovery but I know its close to unlikely.

Day 11:

Today is my first day of eating real foods. I had bacon, and some eggs with cream cooked in bacon fat. What was odd was once I ate the bacon I had no hunger to eat the eggs. I came back several hours later and they were quite good. Had trouble sleeping because I have too much energy. So today I was a little wonked. I don't know if its just one day post fast and having food again or if it will continue. But it looks like I've survived my fast and hopefully with a cleaner liver and pancreas. I will be to the docs in a week so I'll see how my blood work turns out.

Days 12-15 (non fasting)

So Now I'm eating keto. I'm using my keto breath meter just cause its neato and to make sure I'm not falling out of keto. Weight loss seems to be continuing but much slower. A friend said "It's all just water weight" but no the weight has stayed day. I'm up two pounds because now I have food in my intestines again. That's normal. Because I started from a place of extremely sick, I was still dizzy standing. That shouldn't happen to you. But over a few days I get stronger and stronger. Another side effect is it's like I barely need sleep, I'm up and at them at six or eight am. As someone who used to want to sleep till noon, this is a massive change. And it's because I'm sleeping so much better – no more diabetic runs to the bathroom every ten minutes to pee out sugar. I got up about twice to pee, maybe three times. If your young and healthy and non diabetic you have no idea but if your diabetic and got into the big thirst mode and constant peeing, you know the horror. Oh the big thirst is gone. I'm no longer attached to water bottles and guzzling water constantly. That is definitely better. I have no issue at all not eating breads somehow after the fast they just mentally connect with pain and suffering much more. So the hunger for them, unless I'm in a bakery with fresh baked smells, is zero.

I did order a couple of "keto" foods to help me. One was keto granola. There are a few types out there. Makes a nice little snack when you want to nibble. The other I haven't tried yet but its a very very overpriced pancake mix called dees (when I got the pack I paid fourteen dollars for I almost fainted I assumed it was going to be a big bag of mix). And some sugar free carb free syrup. Idea is to make waffles, I know all keto pancakes suck. People make cookies with the mix. Expensive cookies. I'm not a cookies person so I wont.

Bathroom functions all returned in two days of eating. And by two days tummy pains had mostly gone, until I made my instapot chilli with sour cream (my god sooo good). For some reason my tummy felt like a brick was in there for eight hours. But my god soo good. Here is the recipe you can make it in a regular pot, but a instapot just gives you that set it and forget it, it browns the meat on saute mode, pressure cooks it, then I switch it to slow cooker function on low to keep it warm so I don't have to put it in a container until I've eaten another meal of it.

Recipes for KETO

These saved me. I hope you try them.

FatHead Pizza

10oz mozzarella

5oz almond flour

1 egg

1 tsp baking powder

Mozzarella and toppings as you desire

Melt cheese in microwave in 30 second intervals. Mix after each interval.

Add 1 egg and mix with electric mixer.

Mix dry ingredients - 5oz almond flour and 1 tsp baking powder then slowly add to mozzarella and mix in slowly.

Sprinkle counter with a dusting of almond flour.

Knead dough by hand until it resembles regular bread dough. do not over knead as oils will come out.

Roll out onto a baking tray covered in parchment paper and presto - pizza crust. pierce with fork all over.

Precook dough first in the oven at 400 degrees for 8 minutes. Remove from oven

top with a no sugar pizza sauce, mozzarella, and toppings (I'm pepperoni and mushroom and crushed red pepper)

Cook again in the oven for 5-8 more minutes at 400F or until cheese is melted and crust looks browned.

Super Easy Chili

(yes it has beans. But you don't eat many of them each serving)

1 lb the best grass fed beef you can get

2 cans Muir organic fire roasted tomatoes (or any good fire roasted tomatoes)

1 can Goya black beans unrinsed (has to be Goya, they are diff than our bigger American black beans)

3 Anaheim peppers, chopped coarsely

pinch of salt, fresh ground pepper, a good dose of chilli powder (like at least 1 tablespoon)

step 1: brown the beef until no more red and it crumbles. Don't use 85% fast use a leaner grade so you don't have to drain oil

step 2: add all ingredients. If instapot cover and pressure cook on high for 15 mins

step 3: dish up, I put Cholula sauce on top then a big dollop of organic sour cream. But if you don't eat spicy don't and it will be just slight undertones of spice, the anaheims aren't that spicy of a pepper.

It really is an amazing recipe and so simple. I hope you will try it. If just cooking on the stove I would say to simmer for an hour on low heat. This makes about SIX big servings.

Now yes KETO people say no beans. But this recipe needs them. And it wont kill you.

Egg-White Tortillas for Tacos

1/3 cup coconut flour

egg white from 8 eggs (about 1.5 cups)

1 tsp baking powder

pinch of salt

1-2 tablespoons water until soupy

Mix well and should have a thin watery foundation. Put 1/3 cup into a 8" heated skillet and swirl around making it very thin. Once you see it is cooked enough, flip it. Should make a very thin tortilla.

Now you can make tacos again, and enchiladas. Great!

Eating Out Strategies

Rule 1) Forget fast food. It just wont be worth it.

Thai: Order Tom Kha Goong (coconut milk with shrimp soup) but specify NO SUGAR. Or with chicken it's Tom Kha Gai

You can also order a curry again with no sugar. Thai salads with hard boiled egg are good order an extra egg!

Seafood: Get a dozen raw oysters, but ask for melted butter to dip in to up the fat. You can do the same with Lobster. Get a lobster roll sans bun. Dip in melted butter. Or crab. Same same. Expensive but a good treat!

BBQ Places: Nothing wrong with ordering ½ pound of fatty brisket but bring your own NO Sugar BBQ sauce. Because I promise you, the tasty stuff they have is full of sugar.

Of course BBQ places often also have other meats as well – turkey, chicken, etc. All fine but these are lower fat than the fatty brisket (and I think less tasty)

Strategies for a Salad Bar:

You have to do a few things to get a salad to work. Add the hard boiled eggs and bacon if they have it. Top with just balsamic vinegar or use your own brought Olive or Avocado oil made dressing with no sugar. Skip the dressings they have, they are full of sugar.

And finally, for shopping, Costco seems to be stocking a lot of low carb items with much better selection that you might find at your local grocery or Walmart.

The Dangers of Oils and Mayonnaise

Here are the healthy oils:

Natural Animal Fats: Butter (grass fed like KerryGold is best)

Lard, Tallow, Bacon Fat, Suet, etc.

Plant based Oils: Avocado Oil, Olive Oil

For plant based oils, use sparingly and not for cooking

Avocado Oil is good for homemade mayo and 1 or 2 Tablespoons of Extra Virgin Olive oil is ok for on salads.

Then there is coconut oil. The extra virgin is quite expensive. But if you want to deep fry, this is your main choice if you don't have access to large quantities of Beef Fat (tallow) or Lard. It does impart a slight coconuty taste so it's not the best. For french fries, beef fat rules. These should only be for special treats not daily food.

And then there's Mayonnaise. Ugh. There's NOTHING sold in grocery stores that's edible. Even if it says "Avocado oil" in big letters on the front, read the ingredients and it will have forbidden vegetable oils. If you want mayonnaise, get a hand blender (esp one with the flat disk special for making mayo) and the recipe is simple. Crack an egg into a tall narrow container. Turn the hand blender on slow and beat the egg. Then slowly (very!) drizzle in your avocado oil. It should turn white-yellow showing you have successfully emulsified the oil and be like any store bought mayo, but actually with healthier ingredients. Store bought mayo also has SUGAR and in truth, you don't need it. I've always found the high sugar mayos gross anyways.

18 days from the 10 day fast: Update

OK so I passed something very hard and difficult to get out. And then my stomach hard spot was gone. Some gunk stuck there? Most likely. Well I can tell you it was like nothing I've been through before it was pretty rough getting it out. But now My stomach does feel so great.

One other thing that happened is I ate like 2+ cups of blueberries with cream and knocked myself out of ketosis. One cup of blueberries is 12g of carbs so 2+ was closer to 50g of carbs. Ouch. Watch out for blueberries you really have to stick to one cup for a snack with cream. Strawberries and Blackberries and Raspberries have only 6g of carbs so they should be your go to.

And I met the doctor and of course she insisted in the full 300 dollar battery of blood tests. This is going to be interesting. Oddly, I was due my second daily thyroid med dose and without it my heart had gone to 135. eeek. Well that scared them but then I remembered this seemed to be a signal that I needed my thyroid dose. Later that night after the dose, heart rate was back to 90. I think the one number that scares me is the Liver function ALT. I hope it's corrected but I fear it will show still broken. Which means either its PERMANENTLY scarred. In other words I got there too late. OR, I need to do another maybe longer fast to allow more liver recovery. I sorta can guess that my one little fast and 2 weeks of keto isn't enough to reverse it. I will post the scary results here. But I do expect to show a big improvement from my total sick bloodwork.

The last thing to put here is feeling better I finally got to the thai restaurant for my Tom Kha Goong – coconut milk shrimp soup. I asked them to make it without sugar. It came back soo good. Still plenty sweet from the coconut milk. He told me their chili paste had lots of sugar so they cut it way back for my dish. I was so touched. I ate two quarts of this re-feeding soup of life. There was something about it that just felt nourishing. I grabbed the spicy red pepper powder and spiced it up. MMM perfect. Would it toss me out of ketosis? Let's check with the breath meter. Yehp out of ketosis, Oh well it was worth it! You can't beat yourself up too much. A half day fasting and I'll get back into it but today I feel like eating my normal keto breakfast. Eggs with cream, bacon, spinach, and cheese. It's really something I enjoy. Even everyday. I just never seem to tire of it. While the heavier meats seem to be a bit rough on my digestion. I got six big scallops at the store. That's the lunch plan. Then for dinner a hamburger sans bun and a tiny dollop of sugar containing a-1 steak sauce. I know. Not sanctioned. So I have to keep it to just a drop not my normal swimming in it!

Energy is up and doing a grocery store run I almost have the energy for. Still metabolic challenges. I still get a little weak but nothing like before.

Weight has crept UP six pounds. So I've chosen 2 fasting days a week – weds and saturday. Hopefully that will help turn around the weight gain to weight loss. I'm sure it's the fruit that's bonking me out of keto. So once I've eaten the last of the blueberries and strawberries I'm off them. Back to avocado and artichoke hearts for mini meals.

Research References

The most important study for this book is the one that showed that just two weeks of very low calorie input can reduce 80% of liver fat in non-alcoholic fatty liver. That's the basis for the power of the two week or ten day fast. They found

"Mean (+/-SD) LV, VAT/SAT, and body weight decreased significantly (P < 0.001 for all). The degree of LV reduction was directly related to the reduction in relative body weight (r = 0.54, P = 0.001) and initial LV (r = 0.43, P = 0.015). **Eighty percent of the reduction in LV occurred between weeks 0 and 2** (P < 0.001). Reductions in body weight and VAT were uniform over the 12-wk period. Attrition was 14%. Acceptability was adequate but waned over time, and mild transitory side effects occurred.

CONCLUSIONS:

Given the observed early reduction in LV and the progressive reduction in VAT, we suggest that the **minimum duration for a preoperative VLED be 2 wk.** Ideally, the duration should be 6 wk to achieve maximal LV reduction and significant reductions in VAT and body weight without compromising compliance and acceptability."

Here is the study:

> Preoperative weight loss with a very-low-energy diet: **quantitation of changes in liver and abdominal fat by serial imaging.**
>
> Colles SL1, Dixon JB, Marks P, Strauss BJ, O'Brien PE.
>
> Am J Clin Nutr. 2006 Aug;84(2):304-11.

In the Boden study, they performed an in-patient study in obese T2D individuals who were fed a low-carbohydrate (<20 g/day) diet for 2 weeks. Plasma glucose fell from 7.5 to 6.3 mmol/l, haemoglobin A1c decreased from 7.3 to 6.8% and there were dramatic improvements (75%) in insulin sensitivity.

Boden G,Sargrad K,Homko C,Mozzoli M,Stein TP. Effect of a low-carbohydrate diet on appetite, blood glucose levels, and insulin resistance in obese patients with type 2 diabetes.*Ann Intern Med* 2005; **142**: 403–411.

Studies support the long-term efficacy of ketogenic diets in managing complications of type 2 diabetes. Although significant reductions in fat mass often results when individuals restrict carbohydrate, the improvements in glycemic control, hemoglobin A1c and lipid markers, as well as reduced use or withdrawal of insulin and other medications in many cases, occurs before significant weight loss occurs.

Yancy WS Jr,Foy M,Chalecki AM,Vernon MC,Westman EC.A low-carbohydrate, ketogenic diet to treat type 2 diabetes.*Nutr Metab (Lond)*2005;**2**: 34.

Long term studies of the effects of a Ketogenic diet on Diabetes show that it is an effective course of treatment.

Nielsen JV, Joensson EA. Low-carbohydrate diet in type 2 diabetes: Stable improvement of bodyweight and glycemic control **during 44 months** follow-up.*Nutr Metab (Lond)* 2008;**5**: 14.

Scientists at Helmholtz Zentrum München have new information on what happens at the molecular level when we go hungry.

Working with the Deutsches Zentrum für Diabetesforschung (German Center for Diabetes Research -- DZD) and the Deutsches Krebsforschungszentrum (German Cancer Research Center -- DKFZ) they were able to show that upon deprivation of food a certain protein is produced that adjusts the metabolism in the liver. The results are published in the Open Access Journal 'EMBO Molecular Medicine'.

J. Fuhrmeister, A. Zota, T. P. Sijmonsma, O. Seibert, S. Cngr, K. Schmidt, N. Vallon, R. M. de Guia, K. Niopek, M. Berriel Diaz, A. Maida, M. Bluher, J. G. Okun, S. Herzig, A. J. Rose.**Fasting-induced liver GADD45 restrains hepatic fatty acid uptake and improves metabolic health.**EMBO Molecular Medicine, 2016; DOI: 10.15252/emmm.201505801

This next study showed that you can get there and reverse NAFLD if you are able to exercise and restrict calories for a long period of time. Unfortunately, most diabetic patients are very far from being able to do this.Therapeutic effects of restricted diet and exercise in obese patients with fatty liver

TakatoUenoHiroshiSugawaraKoodoSujakuOsamuHashimoto RikoTsujiSeishuTamakiTakujiTorimuraSadatakaInuzukaMichi oSataKyuichiTanikawa

https://doi.org/10.1016/S0168-8278(97)80287-5Get rights and content

There are not as of yet many longer term fasting studies but here is on on shorter term effects on the liver:
"In murine models, time-restricted feeding resets the hepatic circadian clock and enhances transcription of key metabolic regulators of glucose and lipid -homeostasis. Studies of the effect of dawn-to-sunset Ramadan fasting, which is akin to time-restricted feeding model, have also identified significant improvement in body mass index, serum lipid profiles, and oxidative stress parameters. Based on the findings of studies conducted on human subjects, dawn-to-sunset fasting has the potential to be a cost-effective intervention for obesity, metabolic syndrome, and NAFLD. " - Gastroenterology Research and Practice
Volume 2017, Article ID 3932491, 13 pages
https://doi.org/10.1155/2017/3932491 Impact of Time-Restricted Feeding and Dawn-to-Sunset Fasting on Circadian Rhythm, Obesity, Metabolic Syndrome, and Nonalcoholic Fatty

Liver Disease, <u>Ayse L. Mindikoglu</u>,1,2 <u>Antone R. Opekun</u>,2,3 <u>Sood K. Gagan</u>,1 and <u>Sridevi Devaraj</u>4

"Four of 5 post-treatment liver biopsies showed histologic improvements in steatosis (fat in liver)($P=.02$) inflammatory grade ($P=.02$), and fibrosis ($P=.07$). Six months of a low-carbohydrate, ketogenic diet led to significant weight loss and histologic improvement of fatty liver disease. Further research is into this approach is warranted." - <u>Digestive Diseases and Sciences</u>

February 2007, Volume 52, <u>Issue 2</u>, pp 589–593| <u>Cite as</u>

The Effect of a Low-Carbohydrate, Ketogenic Diet on Nonalcoholic Fatty Liver Disease: A Pilot Study, David Tendler, Sauyu Lin, William S. YancyJr., John Mavropoulos, Pam Sylvestre, Don C. Rockey, Eric C. Westman

This is an important study because it shows that you can lose bag4 body fat, but still not reduce fatty liver fat:

"LFAT appears to be related to the amount of fat in the diet rather than the size of endogenous fat depots in obese women. Women with initially high LFAT lost more LFAT by similar weight loss than those with low LFAT, although both groups lost similar amounts of subcutaneous and intra-abdominal fat. These data suggest that LFAT is regulated by factors other than intra-abdominal and subcutaneous fat. Therefore, LFAT does not appear to simply reflect the size of endogenous fat stores."

Effects of Identical Weight Loss on Body Composition and Features of Insulin Resistance in Obese Women With High and Low Liver Fat Content

Mirja Tiikkainen[1],Robert Bergholm[1],Satu Vehkavaara[1],Aila Rissanen[2],Anna-Maija Häkkinen[3],Marjo Tamminen[1],Kari Teramo.Hannele Yki-Järvinen[1]
Diabetes 2003 Mar; 52(3):701-707.https://doi.org/10.2337/diabetes.52.3.701

"In conclusion, the findings that intermittent fasting increases insulin sensitivity on the whole body level as well as in adipose tissue support the view that cycles of feast and famine are important as an initiator of thrifty genes leading to improvements in metabolic function"

Effect of intermittent fasting and refeeding on insulin action in healthy men

Nils Halberg, Morten Henriksen, Nathalie Söderhamn, Bente Stallknecht, Thorkil Ploug
01 DEC
2005https://doi.org/10.1152/japplphysiol.00683.2005

On the relationship between Insulin levels and cancer, in a controlled study, it was found that ketogenic diet and low insulin directly helped slow or reduce cancer tumors.

Fine EJ,Segal-Isaacson CJ,Feinman RD, Herszkopf S,Romano MC,Tomuta N*et al*. Targeting insulin inhibition as a metabolic therapy in advanced cancer: a pilot safety and feasibility dietary trial in 10 patients. *Nutrition* 2012; **28**: 1028–1035.

This is an interesting research article on the beneficial effects of Melatonin on mice and fatty liver. Another article repeated similar results with Hamsters. Hopefully someone will try this with Humans soon but as Melatonin is relatively harmless, I've added it to my dailies. – "The study concluded that melatonin could **improve NAFLD** by decreasing body weight and reduce inflammation in HFD induced obese mice by modulating the MAPK-JNK/P38 signaling pathway."

Melatonin improves non-alcoholic fatty liver disease via MAPK-JNK/P38 signaling in high-fat-diet-induced obese mice.
Sun H1,Wang X1,Chen J2,Song K1,Gusdon AM3,Li L1,Bu L1,Qu S4.

Meringa Leaf has been shown to lower blood glucose in mouse trials. In Mexico and central America where it grows it has been used to treat diabetes. "The consumption of the leaves showed a hypoglycemic effect (< 250 mg/dL in diabetic*M. Oleifera* treated group)"

Effect of Moringa oleifera consumption on diabetic rats

BMC Complement Altern Med. 2018; 18: 127.

Published online 2018 Apr 10. doi: 10.1186/s12906-018-2180-2
PMCID: PMC5894151 PMID: 29636032
A. Villarruel-López,2D. A. López-de la Mora,1O. D. Vázquez-Paulino,2A. G. Puebla-Mora,3Ma R. Torres-Vitela,2L. A. Guerrero-Quiroz,4andK. Nuño⊠ 1

Pills I take daily

People can go crazy with supplements. But Here is what I take based on research.

Meringa (capsules research shows it helps glucose).

Green Tea Concentrate (get the best quality you can)

PQQ (for numbness esp in feet)

Melatonin (helps fatty liver in mice)

Good multivitamin (NOW EVE liquid capsules)

Things I have taken or taken sometimes

Siberian ginseng (general vitality)

Clove (glucose regulation)

Guanabana juice (anti cancer)